Yoga

Essential Yoga Tips and Techniques to Achieve Maximum Stress Relief and Weight Loss

Taylor C. Roldan

Table of Contents

Introduction

If you are looking for one of the few yoga books that will teach you everything you need to know about yoga and weight loss, then Beginners Guide To Yoga Poses is the perfect book for you. Unlike other yoga books, this book contains 30 beginner poses that will not only help you relax and relieve stress, but will help you to lose weight in the process.

You would be surprised how long Yoga has been around. Yoga has been around for nearly 5,000 years. While this practice has roots deeper into our culture than we are even aware of, the truth is that in the United States alone people are not shown the traditional way to do Yoga and instead are fed into doing some kiddie version of it.

Yoga is seen as a practice done on a daily basis to get you into good health and incredible shape. While it is true that numerous Yoga studies have flourished all over the world in the recent years, the sad truth is that these studies often misrepresent what Yoga is truly all about.

Throughout this book I will introduce you to the real world of Yoga, show you the real exercises of Yoga, and teach you all about the real Yoga that most beginners do not know about. I urge you to use every technique I teach you in this book, especially if you are looking to lose weight or just looking to get in the best shape of your life. Everything that you find in this book will benefit you in the long run.

I want to sincerely thank you for purchasing it, and I hope you enjoy it.

Let's get started!

Chapter 1: The Basics of Yoga

So, to start, what exactly is Yoga? When it is defined, Yoga is simply the collection of both physical and spiritual practices that are aimed at enhancing the state of the body, mind, and spirit. The main goal of yoga is to help achieve a state of balance within yourself and to ultimately bring enlightenment to your life.

There are many different paths of yoga. The one that many people in the United States are familiar with is known as Hatha Yoga. This path of yoga is most commonly referred to as the "forceful" or physical path of Yoga. In Eastern countries, the different paths of yoga that are practiced focus primarily on meditation, participating in selfless services, and complete devotion.

While all of the different paths of yoga use different approaches and technique, they are all supposed to lead to the same goal of unifying people together and enlightening one's life. Even though the goal of yoga is somewhat lofty at times, its very essence is rooted in practicality and science. While Yoga does use spiritual techniques to help bring enlightenment to a person, it is not a religious practice.

The History of Yoga

The origin of Yoga is mostly obscured because of its secrecy throughout the ages and its resilience throughout time. The earliest mention of this practice was found in the form of transcriptions laid out on extremely fragile palm leaves. These leaves were damaged over time, lost, or completely destroyed. While the evidence of this practice has been lost throughout the ages, many scholars believe that it originated around 5,000 years ago, but there are many experts out there that believe this practice can be as old as 10,000 years.

The origin of this practice was originally developed by a civilization in the Northern part of India known as the Indus-Sarasvati civilization. When this practice was first introduced it was used in the context of a guru-disciple relationship and helped to strengthen the bonds between the two. In those times, people practiced Yoga to seek to diminish or put a stop to the vitality of their body in order to control the unnatural desires that make us all human. These human obstacles were viewed as obstacles in the way of liberation back then.

That is when many yoga masters of the time began to see the body as a vehicle of transformation rather than the hindrance of it and then created a system that was designed to use practices to help balance and energize the body and help it prepare for liberation. This philosophy became known as Tantra Yoga, which eventually became the precursor for Hatha Yoga which the form and practice that you see most commonly in the United States today.

Around the 1920's and 1930's, Hatha Yoga was most used and promoted in India through a variety of different Yoga masters such as Swami Sivananda and T. Krishnamacharya. Sivananada was a prolific yoga master and wrote near 200 books on the very subject. He even started numerous popular yoga centers across the globe.

In Depth Look at Hatha Yoga

As I mentioned before, Yoga that moved to the west and into countries like the United States is often referred to as Hatha Yoga. The word Hatha literally translates to the sun and the moon. This type of yoga is described to be used as a way to attain the union between the body, mind, and spirit through the use of asanas or yoga postures, pranayama or yoga breathing, mudra or body gestures, and shatkarma or internal cleansing.

The practices and exercises of this type of yoga were designed in such a way that they are meant to help the body to purify itself and to activate the kundalini of energy molecules inside of the body. It is important to keep in mind that modern day hatha yoga does not use many of these practices and simply focuses primarily on the physical yoga postures themselves.

When you look back at yoga history as a whole, this form of yoga is a fairly recent technique and was originally developed from Tantra Yoga.

The people behind this type of yoga embraced the beauty of the physical body and used it as a means to achieve enlightenment by developing the spiritual connections between the mind and body.

Chapter 2: The Different Styles of Yoga and Their Benefits

Remember, if you are interested in yoga and want to try it out for yourself, there are many different types, styles, and schools of yoga out there so you can find the perfect one for you. Once you begin yoga, I highly recommend that you start off with a list of the things that you want to achieve using yoga whether that is to do it into some smaller clothes, to relieve some stress, or to meditate.

In this chapter I want to discuss the different styles of yoga and the benefits of doing it so you can see whether or not yoga is for you.

Type #1: Anusara

This type of yoga was originally developed in 1997 by an American man by the name of John Friend. Anusara literally means "To step into divine will" and it was founded on the premise of the fact that we are all filled with some form of inner goodness. This type of yoga was aimed to teach students to let this inner goodness shine through to the outside so that they can reach that feeling of enlightenment.

The yoga classes that teach this kind of yoga have been known to be quite rigorous on the students, pushing them to the limit both mentally and physically. Not only is it very draining on the mind and body, but it is very satisfying as well.

Type #2: Ashtanga

This type of yoga was founded on very ancient principles, but it was not introduced or made popular in the West until the 1970's by a person names Pattie Jois. This tough and rigorous yoga style has its students go through a series of different postures and with each posture they go into, they are supposed to breathe a certain way. This is one of most demanding exercises known in the yoga world and it is one that will get you sweating right away.

This is the best type of yoga for those who are either ex-athletes or those who are looking for a mental and physically exerting exercise that will push them to their very limit. The one characteristic that sticks out with this type of yoga is that the same positions are used in exactly the same order every time.

Type #3: Bikram

This type of yoga was originally developed by a person by the name of Bikram Choudhry. This is certainly one type of yoga that most people do not forget for long. The classes that are usually held for this type of exercise are held in rooms that are heated up to 105 degrees and with a humidity level up to 40%. In these specially heated and humidified room students are asked to work through nearly 26 different poses, making students sweat much more than they have ever sweat before.

Why do teachers expose students to these extreme temperatures? Well, for starters, it is well know that whenever we sweat, it helps to eliminate harmful toxins from the body. So, the more that you sweat, the healthier you will be in the long run.

Out of all of the different types of yoga, the Bikram style is actually one of the easiest to find in terms of classes. It is also the strictest of the types, as students MUST follow the sequence of different yoga postures to the T, exactly as the founder developed it.

Type #4: Hatha

This is one style that we have already discussed in some detail in this book. This type is considered to be the generic form of yoga today and primarily teaches students how to go into basic physical poses. This type of yoga is so common today is that nearly every type of class that can be found in the West today teaches Hatha yoga.

This type of yoga introduces the basic yoga postures that are considered to be the most basic in yoga today. With this type I want you to know that you will probably not be able to break out in much of a sweat. However, you will benefit with an increase in flexibility and you will feel much more relaxed the more you do it. I highly recommend the poses within this type if you are looking for the perfect way to wind down at night.

Type #5: Iyengar

The person who developed this style of yoga goes by the name of B.K.S Iyengar. Unlike the other styles, this particular style is all about finding the proper alignment in every pose that you do in a meticulous manner. When you find studios that teach and specialize in this type of yoga, you will find that they are equipped with many different props to help with this meticulous alignment such as blocks, chairs, straps, blankets, and a rope wall.

While this may seem like it is one of the most active types of yoga today, it is not meant to get your heart racing. On the contrary, it is meant to challenge your mind and your body with every pose that you get yourself into.

To add to this type, the instructors who teach it are required to undergo extensive and comprehensive training into the different poses. This type of yoga is ideal for those who have suffered an injury in the past and that need to go through physical therapy. This is certainly the type that will heal your mind and your body together.

Type #6: Vinyasa

The word Vinyasa literally means "to flow" and for this particular reason, the Vinyasa yoga style is most famous for its fluid like and intense poses. The poses are well choreographed when you transition from pose to pose and most of the classes that teach this style are often blaring with music to help enhance the transitions into the various poses.

The Vinyasa style of yoga is similar to the Ashtanga style in terms of intensity, but you will find that no two Vinyasa yoga classes are exactly the same. This particular style is well suited for people who want challenge the limits of their body and mind, but who are not a fan of routines. This is for people who like to switch things up every once in a while.

Type #7: Kundalina

This style of yoga refers to the Chakra energy root, which is located near the region of the base of the backbone. This type of style is meant to work out the core areas of your body with intense poses that are unlike other styles of yoga.

Type #8: Ananda

The Ananda yoga style is very different from any of the previous yoga poses that we have discussed. This style is meant to provide you with more than just the development of your physical body. Rather it is a tool that is used for eliminating tension and stress as well as increasing the bond to spiritual health.

This style of yoga was developed sometime in the 1960's by a person by the name of Swami Kriyananda. The main reason why this particular style is much different from the other types of yoga is that while you do the various poses, you must do so while silently saying affirmations. This style is mostly focused on breathing in a controlled way, using the proper alignment as you go through the various poses and transitioning smoothly in each and every pose that you go into.

With the various different types of yoga that are available today, it is important that you embrace whichever type that you choose to try. Each type will come with its own unique benefits and in the next part we will explore the benefits of yoga and how you can become a much happier and healthier person by doing yoga.

How Will Yoga Benefit You?

Yoga, as a whole, can offer various benefits to your entire body. Just think about it: today we expose ourselves to various diseases, whether they be physical or mental. Yoga is very beneficial as it can help you not only clear your mind, but allow you to achieve what is truly important in life as well: good health and true happiness.

There are a variety of benefits to yoga and in this section we will explore those benefits.

1. Can Help Improve Mental Health

As many people are aware, with today's lifestyle it can be really hard to achieve optimum physical health and mental health at the same time. Yoga can certainly help with this. The core of yoga is about using proper breathing techniques along with proper postures to help enhance the health of your body. When you learn how to breathe properly, this allows the cells within your body to get the right amount of oxygen that they need for longer periods of time.

When you get the perfect amount of oxygen, your brain will benefit by improving your overall cognitive performance. By having more cognitive performance, you will have the ability to have more clear and concise thoughts that could improve your overall self-esteem and self-confidence.

This can help exceptionally with children who suffer from a variety of mental disorders such as ADD or attention deficit disorder or ADHD. Yoga can also be beneficial to those who are suffering from various mood swings, depression, and anxiety. Yoga is meant to help keep the mind calm and to reduce the amount of stress you are suffering from.

2. Can Help Boost Your Overall Strength

Have you ever come home after a long day at work, crashed onto your sofa, and felt way too tired to even lift the remote for your TV? Many of us go through this on a daily basis and this is not something that occurs simply because we are tired. This occurs due to lack of inner strength.

There are various yoga poses available that can help enhance the strength within each and every one of us. Generating this inner strength is important to help us accomplish even the most basic of tasks on a daily basis and to avoid injuries that we can sustain from simply not paying attention.

Yoga is meant to increase the amount of energy you have, as well as boost your overall vitality. Yoga is highly beneficial to those who are in their senior years simply because seniors today require much more energy to do some of the same activities that we consider to be easy.

3. Can Help Improve Your Flexibility

Many people today have the false pretense that in order to do yoga, you have to be flexible, when it fact it is actually the other way around. In order to become more flexible, you should do yoga. When you do yoga, it involves a lot of exercising and stretching throughout the entire process which has been shown to improve your overall flexibility while reducing the amount of pain that you feel.

One thing about yoga that most people are unaware of is that it can also help your entire body to align itself on its own by giving you posture that is considered good. It helps to work out both your muscles and soft tissues within your body while reduce the amount of lactic acid that accumulates within your body. It also works by increasing your range of motion, which can lead to much better lubrication and mobility of all of your joints.

4. Can Help Improve Cardiovascular Health

We all know how important our hearts really are. Without our hearts, we wouldn't be living. It's as simple as that. Developing a healthy heart system is necessary to prevent harmful and even fatal diseases, such as strokes, heart attacks, and high blood pressure. All of these diseases are caused by not only a poor family medical history, but by negative thinking, an improper lifestyle, and a poor diet.

Yoga can help in this instance by helping to control all of the unhealthy and negative chemical processes within the body and providing the body with a fresh source of oxygen. This fresh source of oxygen can help prevent the negative emotions that you may be feeling and enhance the general well-being of your mental state of mind.

5. Can Help Alleviate Sever Joint and Arthritis Pain

There are many people who suffer from inflammation and stiffness of their joints. When this happens, most people avoid exercising themselves. Yoga can help with this inflammation as it helps to prevent these kinds of ailments by helping to tone of the muscles within the body and by loosening the joints. When you use yoga, you have to go through a series of poses that will strengthen and stretch the muscles within your body. It also helps to enhance the blood flow going to the joints, muscles and tissues of your body that are stiff or sore. What does this mean? It means that your joints will be less painful and that you will be able to move more freely without any fear of pain.

6. Can Help To Prevent Respiratory Problems

There are many different yoga poses that, when done correctly, can act as a way to control a variety of respiratory problems, such as chronic asthma. How is this possible? When you practice yoga, it helps to increase the capacity and stamina of your lungs and eliminates the stress on the passageways of your lungs.

7. Can Help Improve Your Memory

Yoga, when used correctly, is meant to help you to focus on meditation and to improve your concentration. This can help you to hold in more information and to increase your memory for longer periods of time. There are various breathing techniques, meditating exercises, and concentration that you use when you do yoga. This can lead to an improved blood flow to your brain, which enhances the ability for you to accept and retain more information. If you are looking to stop suffering from short term memory loss, this is something that you should certainly try.

8. Can Help You Lose Weight

Losing weight is something that nearly all of us want to do. Obesity in many people today can be due to a variety of different reasons such as eating out of stress, hormonal imbalances, digestive imbalances, bad eating habits, and lack of exercise. By doing yoga, your body will take in even more energy, increase your metabolism, and break down fat cells. With the improved breathing that comes with doing yoga it helps to stimulate your abdominal organs to improve your digestion.

9. Can Help Combat the Effects of Ageing

Yoga helps to refresh both your mind and body and helps you to approach your life in a more positive and stress-free way. When you combine this new way of thinking with the flexibility, mental capacity, and enhanced fitness that yoga brings you, you will be practically glowing with new youth. If you want to feel and look younger, yoga is certainly one way to do it.

Now that you understand what the benefits of yoga are, the next thing for you to do is to begin practicing it. I will teach you how to do just that in the next few chapters so you can feel all these benefits for yourself.

Chapter 3: Common Beginner Mistakes to Avoid

As a newcomer to yoga, you may be a bit anxious about some of the mistakes that you can possibly make while sitting in a yoga class or upon a yoga mat. The very first lesson that you need to teach yourself is not to worry so much about the kinds of mistakes that you will make. The more mistakes that you make, the more you will learn in the process. However, if this is something that you cannot stop worrying about, in this chapter I will list out a few common mistakes that every beginner should avoid making.

Mistake #1: Not Knowing What the Need Is

This is where many beginners keep making mistakes, except of course for those who approach their yoga instructor with a specific health condition in mind. The truth of the matter is that many people enroll in yoga classes without being fully aware of why they need to do so.

There are many styles of yoga out there and you need to choose the right one that will be the best fit for you. When enrolling in yoga classes, take into account your age, how flexible you are, what your health condition is, and what level of passion you have for it.

The best advice that I can give you for this is to talk to your yoga instructor ahead of time and they will guide you appropriately.

Mistaking #2: Comparing Too Much

As much as you may be tempted to do so, try to avoid comparing yourself to others. While the person on the mat next to you may be a bit more flexible than you are, this should not concern you too much. The more you compare yourself to others, the more inferior you will feel about yourself. Do yourself a favor and just strive to do your best. Before you know it, you may outperform all of your classmates.

Mistake #3: Not Breathing In Coordination

This is yet another common mistake that many newcomers to yoga make: breathing. There are many "newbies" that tend to hold their breath while they are in a certain pose and there are others who do not coordinate their breath in time with their movements. The important thing is that you focus on your inhalation and exhalation as you go through a pose. This will help you to improve your pose as well as keep your mind in tune with your movements.

Mistake #4: Pushing Too Hard

One of the most common scenarios that many beginners find themselves in is that they become too excited to try out some new poses and they try to achieve perfection right from the moment that they start. The only thing that will come of this is that you may lose interest in yoga that moment you find it too difficult to achieve the results that you want. Not only will this infuriate you but it may lead to a yoga injury.

While I know both of these possibilities are not desirable in any regard, the only thing that I can recommend is that you evaluate how flexible you are and try to work out a plan to improve your form so that you can succeed in the long run.

Mistake #5: Not Planning

In order to advance into yoga further, the best thing that you can do is to plan each and every yoga session that you have and take into account a variety of factors such as flexibility, your overall health, and, of course, the time that you have. If you do not have a plan, expect enthusiasm to wane after time.

When you have a plan in place you will commit yourself to following it through completely without coming up with any excuses and this will lead to your producing amazing results. This should be enough in itself that you will ultimately practice yoga regularly. In order to succeed, you have to plan. It is as simple as that.

Chapter 4: Thirty Yoga Poses for Beginners

As a beginner in yoga, I highly recommend that you start off with a few simple poses so you don't overstress yourself. In this chapter, you will find 30 of the simplest yoga poses aimed at giving you all the benefits that yoga has to offer. I suggest that you do not push yourself too hard with these exercises. I know how tempting it can be to get all of these poses perfect each and every time, but since you are just starting out, I wouldn't worry about that. With practice, you will be able to perfect these poses in no time.

Pose 1. The Half Wheel Pose

This is one yoga pose that can be used to alleviate symptoms associated with menopause. It can also help to aid digestion by stimulating your abdominal organs to function much better. If you are looking for a way to trim some excess belly fat, this is certainly the pose to do.

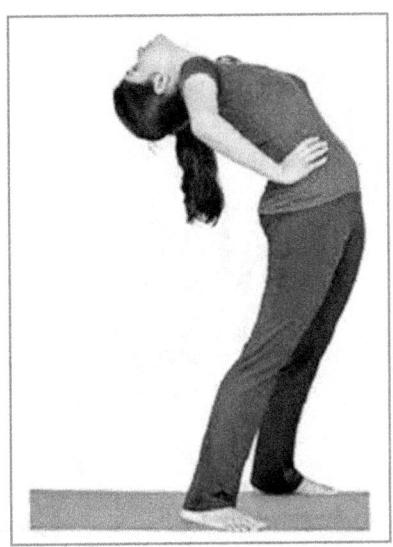

How To Do This Pose:

- Stand straight up and place your feet together. Then place your hands on your waist.
- As you inhale, bend backwards. Make sure that you do not bend your knees as you do this.
- Return to the starting position and repeat.
- Continue to do this pose for a duration of 20 seconds.

Pose 2. The Lotus Pose

This is perhaps the best pose to use for meditation purposes. This pose will help you to keep your mind calm and will help you relax your nervous system. It will also stretch out your spine and strengthen your hips.

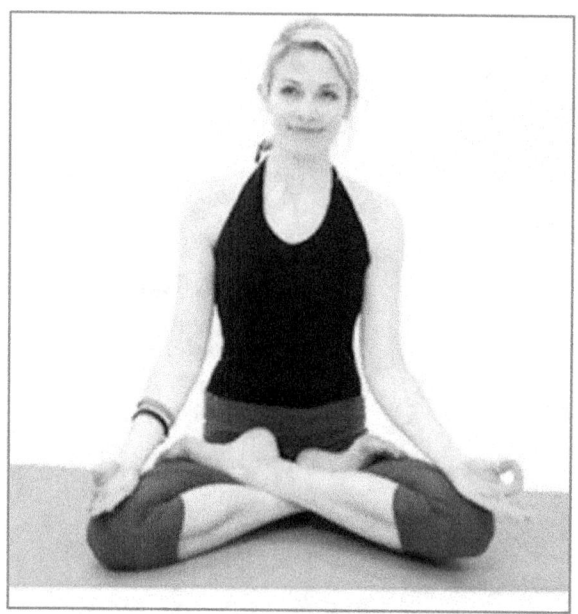

How To Do This Pose:

- Sit on the floor with your legs stretched forward in front of you.
- Make sure that you keep your back straight.
- Then bend your right leg and right foot towards you. Then place your right foot on your left thigh by using your right heel to bring it closer to your body.
- Next bend your left leg to place your left foot over your right thigh. Do this as you did your right foot and leg.
- Stretch both of your arms out and place them upon your knees. Make sure that your palms are facing upward.

- Start assuming Chin Mudhra. To do this, bring the tip of your index finger to the tip of your thumb, but make sure that you keep the remaining fingers stretched out.
- Now inhale and exhale slowly.
- The Duration of This Exercise: 1 Minute
- If you are suffering from ankle and knee injuries, use caution when practicing this pose. The moment that you master this pose, you can stay in this pose for up to an hour. Remember, it is great for meditation.

Pose 3. The Easy Pose

This pose has its name for a reason. This pose is recommended for those who have difficulty doing the lotus pose. If you feel comfortable doing this pose, then I recommend giving the Lotus pose a try. Similar to the first, this pose is highly recommended if you are looking to do some meditation.

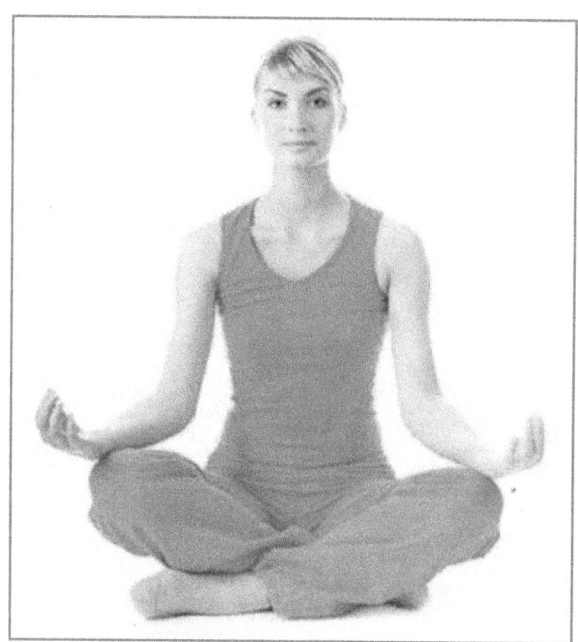

How To Do This Pose:

- Sit on a yoga mat with your legs stretched out in front of you and with your back perfectly straight.
- Then bend your leg in order to place your right foot just below your left thigh.
- Next bend your left leg and place your left foot just below your right thigh.

- With your back perfectly straight, place your palms upon your knees and assume the Chin Mudhra that was discussed in the first pose.
- Then inhale and exhale as slowly as possible.
- Do this exercise for at least 1 minute

Pose 4. The Twisted Pose

This pose is highly recommended for those who are currently treating diabetes. This pose, when done correctly helps to make your spine more flexible and helps to reduce any excess fat that may be in your midsection.

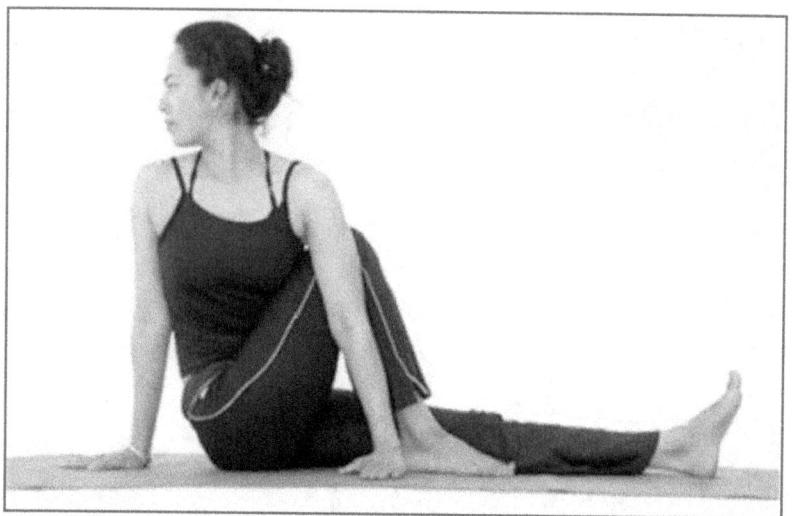

How To Do This Pose:

- Sit down on a yoga mat with your legs stretched out in front of you.
- While you exhale, fold in your right leg and place your right foot near the inside of your left knee.
- Then while inhaling place your right hand against the back of your right buttocks, making sure that your fingers point outwards. Make sure that you maintain some space between your butt and your hand for comfort.
- Bring in your left hand over your right knee, making sure to hold in the ankle of your right leg. Don't hesitate to place your palm by your right leg for comfort.
- Then exhale and twist your spine while you do this.

- Return to your previous position and repeat using your opposite leg.
- Do this exercise for no more than 30 seconds.

Pose 5. The Head to Knee Pose

The purpose of this pose is to stretch out your spine, your shoulders, and your hamstrings in a non-painful way. This pose will help aid in digestion and to close off your mind whenever you need a break from the harshness of reality.

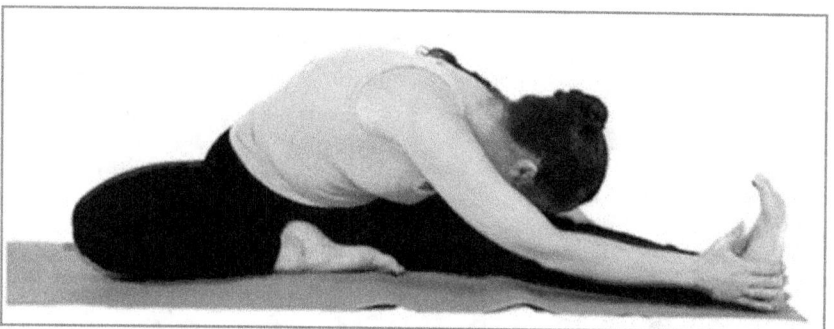

How To Do This Pose:

- Sit on a yoga mat and place your legs stretched out in front of you. Make sure that you keep your back perfectly straight and your feet placed close together.
- Then bend your right knee in order to bring your heel closer to your inner area.
- Then place your right foot beside the inside of your left thigh. Make sure that you let your right knee remain on the floor.
- As your inhale, lift both of your hands sideways and bring them over your head.
- As you exhale bend yourself forward and hold onto your toes of your left leg, which is stretched out.
- While you do this, allow your abdomen to sit on your left thigh while your forehead rests on your left knee. Make sure that you do not bend this stretched out leg.
- Return to your beginning position and repeat the process using your other leg.

- Do this exercise for no more than 20 seconds on each leg.
- If you suffer from severe knee pain or diarrhea, I highly recommend that you stay away from this pose.

Pose 6. The Seated Forward Bend Pose

This pose, when done correctly, will stretch out your entire spine and body, from the base of your neck down to your feet. This pose will help to stimulate the overall performance of all of your internal abdominal organs. It will also help reduce some of that belly fat you are looking to get rid of while keep your mind calm. This is one of the most popular poses used when students are looking to stimulate their Kundalini power.

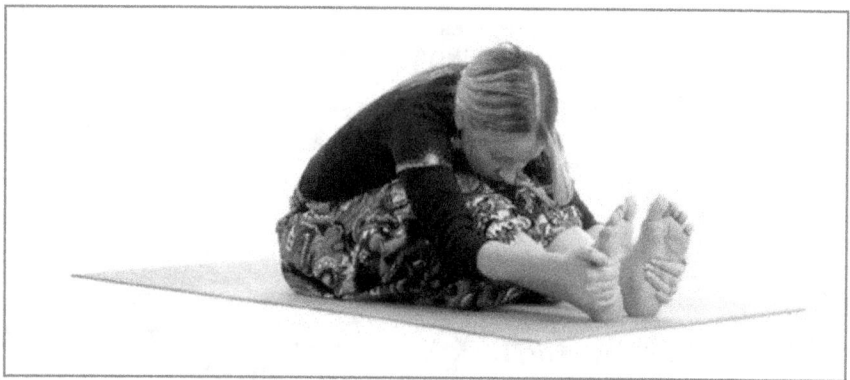

How To Do This Pose:

- Sit down on a yoga mat and stretch out your legs in front of you. Make sure that you keep your back perfectly straight.
- Allow your legs to be closer to your body while your toes are pointed up.
- As you inhale, lift your hands sideways and bring them up over your head.
- Then bend your body forward and reach for your toes as you exhale.
- Hold onto your feet and stretch out your entire spine. Place your chest upon your thighs and rest your forehead upon your knees. If you can stretch out really well, then try to place your forehead as

close as you can to your feet. Make sure that you do not bend your knees.

- Return to your beginning position and lift up your arms to help straighten your back. Place your palms beside you on the floor by both sides of your body.
- Do this exercise for no more than 20 seconds
- I highly suggest that you do not push yourself too hard as your reach for your toes. This is not a competition. Go about it gently and hold onto your legs if you cannot reach your toes. If you are a person suffering from sciatic nerve pain or slipped discs, please refrain from trying this pose.

Pose 7. The Thunderbolt Pose

This is the one pose that you can do after you have finished eating. The reason why this pose is one of the few that is recommended to do immediately after eating is because it helps to aid in digestion. Like the rest, this pose is another that is recommend for mediation as well.

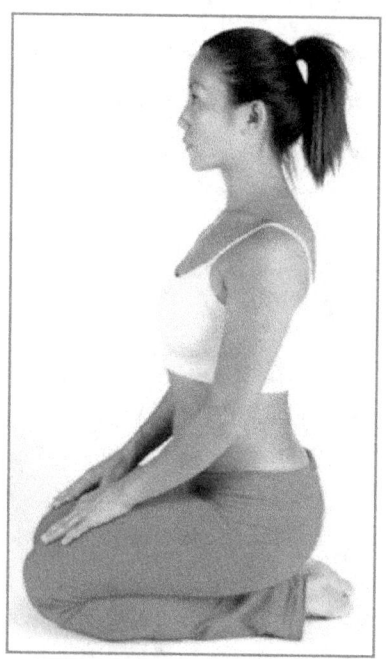

How To Do This Pose:

- The first thing that you will want to do is kneel down on your yoga mat, making sure that you let your thighs touch together.
- Then space out your heels, making sure that your big toes remain in contact. When you do this alignment, envision the letter V.
- Then place your butt onto the space that is between your heels, making sure that you keep your back perfectly straight.
- Place your palms upon your knees, making sure that you do not bend your elbows.

- As you do this, inhale and exhale as slowly as possible.
- Do this exercise for no more than a minute.
- You can increase the duration of this exercise by up to 5 minutes the moment you are comfortable with the pose itself. If you suffer from knee pain or sever knee conditions, I highly recommend that you avoid doing this pose.

Pose 8. The Hero Pose

Just as the name implies this yoga pose will make you feel like a hero. This pose, when done correctly, will help you to strengthen your joints in your knees. It helps to stretch out your thighs and relive any aches or pains that you may be feeling. This pose also helps to cure digestions and is one of the most effective poses to do if you are suffering from menopausal symptoms.

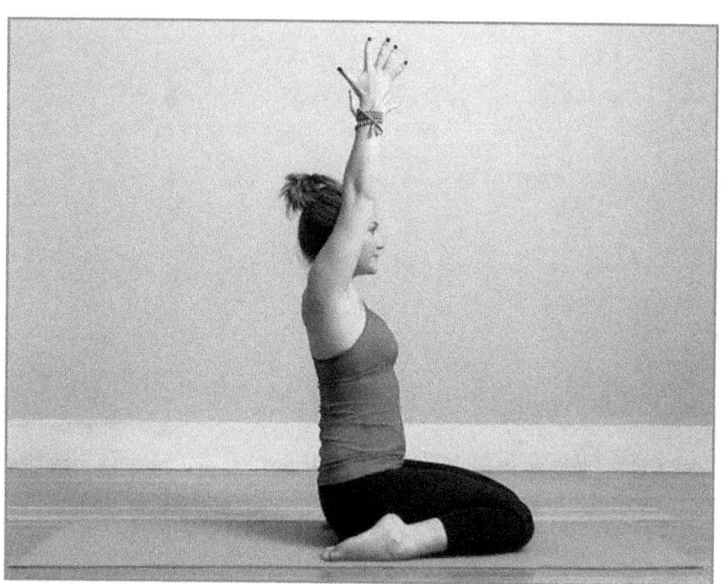

How To Do This Pose:

- To do this pose you will first have to assume the Thunderbolt Pose that was described in this chapter earlier.
- Then space out your feet, making sure that you keep your thighs close together. Next sit down on the space that is between your feet.
- As you inhale, lift your hands sideways. Exhale and stretch out your hands above your head, making sure to lock your fingers together, and move your palms upwards.

- Return to the beginning position and get back into your thunderbolt pose. Make sure that you stretch out your legs in front of you.
- Do this exercise for a duration of 20 seconds.
- If you are suffering from knee problems that are considered severe, then I recommend that you refrain from doing this pose.

Pose 9. The Camel Pose

This pose is perfect for those who suffer from a variety of respiratory issues. This pose works specifically by improving your lung capacity and thereby helping you to breathe much easier and much better. This pose will also help to relieve pain in your upper back area, relieve stress that you may have in your neck, and also help to stimulate the nerves along your spine.

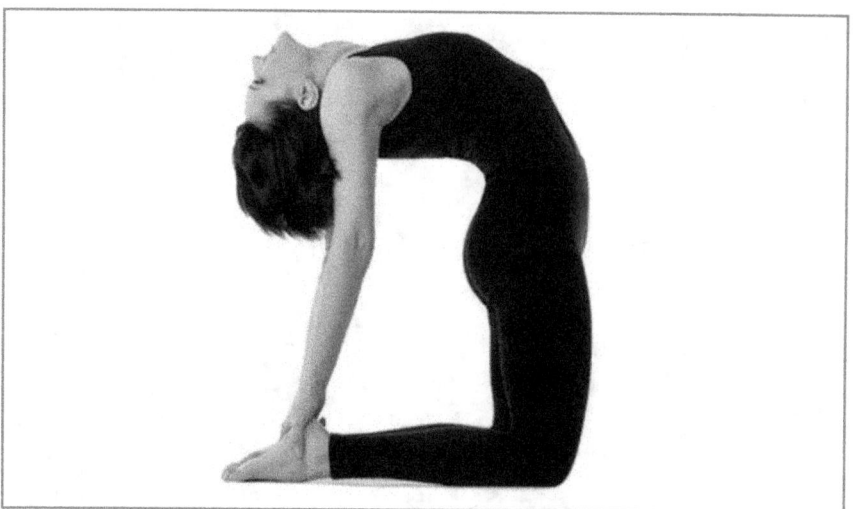

How To Do This Pose:

- The first thing that you will want to do is kneel down on your yoga mat. Then space out your legs, making sure that you maintain a good hip width distance between them.
- Then inhale and as you do so, lift your hands over your head.
- Bend backwards and hold your ankles gently using your hands. Exhale as you do this. Feel free to place your palms on your feet as well.
- Make sure that your hips are in line with your needs. This will give you a good arch for your back.

- Return to the first position simply by releasing your ankles and by making sure that your back is completely straight.
- Do this exercise for no more than 20 seconds.
- If you suffer from chronic migraines, back ailments, low blood pressure, or high blood pressure, I highly recommend that you avoid trying out this pose for yourself.

Pose 10. The Popular Downward Dog Pose

This is one pose that is popularly known among people who don't do yoga because of its awkwardness. Regardless, this is one of the best poses if you are looking for anti-ageing solutions. This pose can be used to improve a variety of issues such as low immunity, issues related to menopause, and for relieving stress.

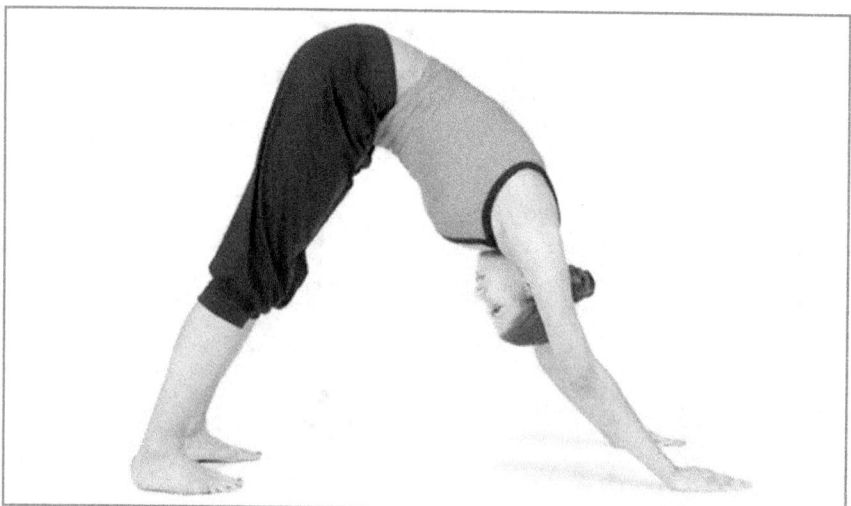

How To Do This Pose:

- The first thing that you will want to do is to get down on floor on all four limbs. Make sure that both your hands and your hips are aligned with your shoulders. Keep your feet at least hip width apart from one another.
- Inhale deeply.
- As you exhale, lift your body up by placing your palms and feet firmly onto the ground. Make sure that as you do this that you do not bend either your knees or your elbows.
- Make sure that your head remains in line with your outstretched hands. At this point, your hips should be raised as high as you can

raise them. Your body will resemble an inverted V at this point as well.

- Return to your first position and simply place your knees on the ground first.
- The duration of this pose should last no longer than a full minute.
- If you are suffering from chronic back issues and high blood pressure, I recommend not trying this pose for yourself.

Pose 11. The Child Pose

If you are looking for a yoga pose that will help you to improve circulation throughout your entire body, this is certainly the pose for you. This pose will help improve circulation from your head to your toes and calm your mind in the process. This pose, while stretching out your spine, is an effective pose to alleviate both neck and shoulder pain.

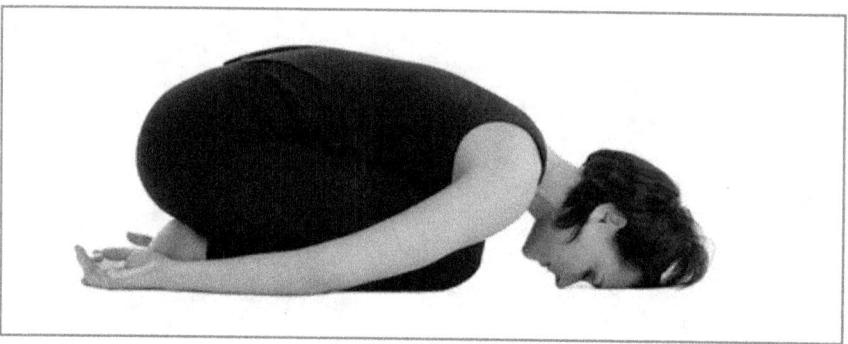

How To Do This Pose:

- The first thing that you will want to do is to get into the Thunderbolt Pose.
- Then as you inhale, bring your arms up over your head.
- As you exhale, bend your body forward and place your forehead gently onto the floor.
- With your body still in this position, stretch out your arms in front of you and then place them by your sides with the palms of your hands facing upwards.
- Return to the thunderbolt position.
- Do this exercise for a duration of no more than 30 seconds.
- If you are suffering from chronic knee and ankle pain and have high blood pressure, I encourage that you refrain from doing this pose.

Pose 12. The Yoga Mudra Pose

This pose is designed in such a way that it will help to tone up your abdominal muscles as well as enhance the performance of all of your abdominal organs. This is one of the poses that are effective if you are suffering from severe constipation.

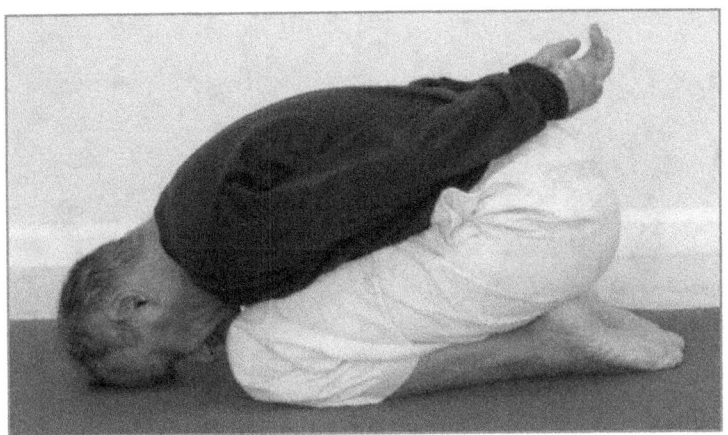

How To Do This Pose:

- The first thing that you will want to do is kneel down on the floor. Sit back and rest your buttocks on your heels.
- Then bring your hands behind your back, making sure that you hold your left wrist with your right hand.
- Exhale and as you do so bend your body forward and place your forehead gently onto the floor. Make sure that you do not lift your buttocks in the process.
- Return to the Padmasana position and repeat.
- Do this pose for a duration of no more than 30 seconds.
- If you suffer from severe knee and hip pain, you should avoid practicing this pose.

Pose 13. The Classic Cobbler's Pose

The cobbler's pose if one of the best poses to use if you are pregnant and are expected to deliver soon. This pose will help to ensure a much easier delivery while also help to combat aging. It can also be used to combat incontinence.

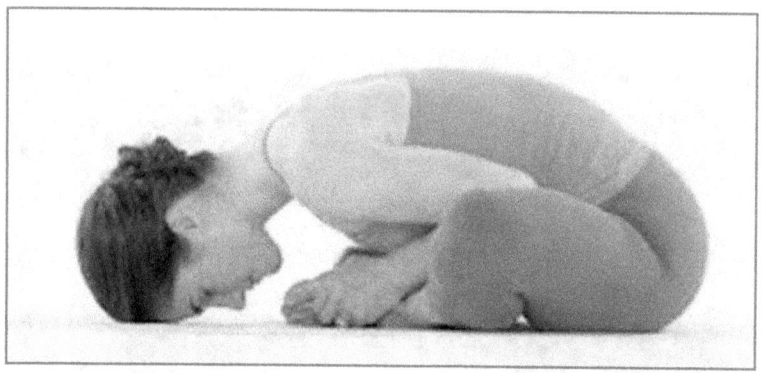

How To Do This Pose:

- The first thing that you will want to do is to sit down on the floor with your legs stretched out in front of you.
- As you inhale deeply bring both of your feet towards your body and place them together. Make sure that you keep your legs on the floor at all times.
- Hold onto your toes with your hands and at the same time stretch out your hands in front of you. Make sure that you keep your palms down.
- Exhale deeply and bend your body forward to place your forehead gently onto the floor. If you are pregnant, do not force yourself to reach the floor. Just do as much as your body will allow you to do.
- Return to your beginning position and repeat.
- Do this pose for a duration of 60 seconds.
- If you suffer from chronic knee issues, do not do this pose at all.

Pose 14. The Bridge Pose

This pose is designed in such a way that it will help to strengthen your spine and your back. It will also help to aid in treating depression and alleviate pain in your neck as well.

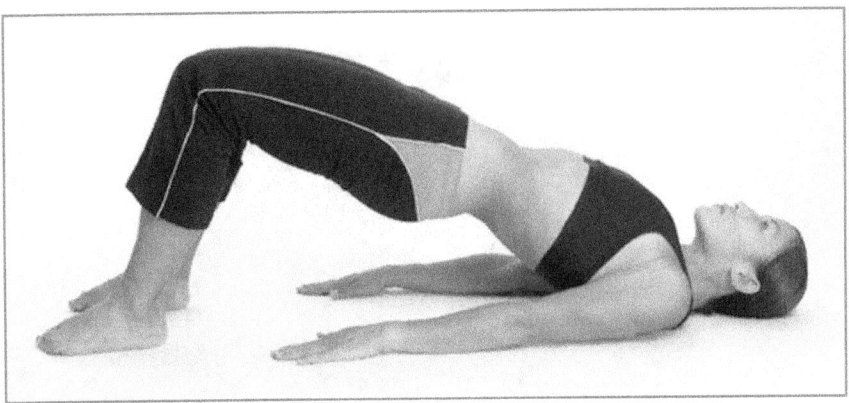

How To Do This Pose:

- Lie down on the floor on your yoga mat. Make sure you lie down flat on your back.
- Place your arms by your sides, making sure that your palms are facing downwards.
- Bend your knees and then place your feet on the ground. Make sure that your feet are perpendicular to your knees. Your feet should also be placed apart, about hips width in distance between them.
- While your hands are planted firmly on the ground, inhale and lift your hips off of the ground. Raise them as high as you possibly can.
- Return to your beginning position as you exhale.
- Continue with this exercise for a duration of 30 seconds.
- If you suffer from chronic back pain, chronic migraines, low blood pressure, or high blood pressure, I highly recommend that you avoid doing this pose.

Pose 15. The Half-Plough Pose

The half-plough pose is used in such a way that it will tone your abdominal muscles and stimulate abdominal function performance at the same time. This pose will also help to tone your thigh muscles as well.

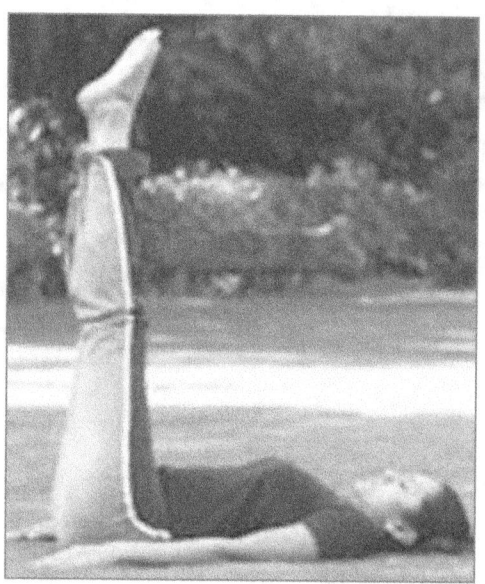

How To Do This Pose:

- Lie down flat on your back upon a yoga mat. Make sure that you place your hands down at your sides as well. Inhale.
- As you exhale raise both of your legs off of the floor and place them at a 90 degree angle. Make sure that you do not bend your knees at all.
- Return to your beginning position and repeat.
- Continue this exercise for a duration of 20 seconds.

Pose 16. The Wind Relieving Pose

This pose is one of the best poses for treating excess flatulence and improving digestion. This is one pose that can help alleviate symptoms of rheumatoid arthritis.

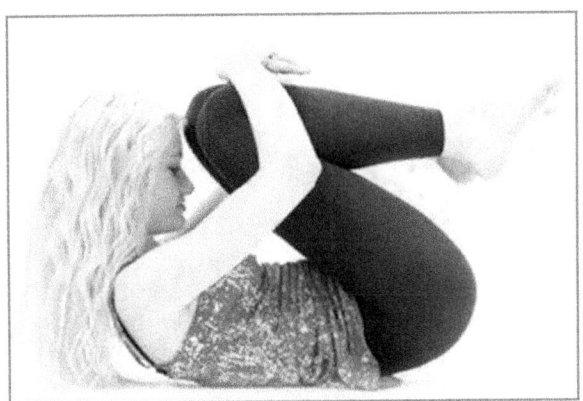

How To Do This Pose:

- Lie down flat on your yoga mat with your hands placed at your sides. Then raise both of your legs off of the floor.
- As you exhale, fold your legs and place your thighs onto your abdomen. Using your palms, gently press your legs down until your knees are close to your chin. Make sure that you do not lift your back at all. Feel free to lock your fingers just over your legs below your knees in order to bring them down further.
- Then lift your head until your chin or your forehead is touching your knees.
- Return to your beginning position and repeat.
- Do this pose for a duration of 20 seconds.
- If you are suffering from severe neck pain, make sure that you do not lift your head or put too much strain on your neck. If you suffer from high blood pressure, make sure that you do not lift up your head as well.

Pose 17. The Boat Pose

This pose is used primarily to treat indigestion. It will also help to stimulate the performance of your liver, kidneys, and pancreas while trimming your belly fat in the process.

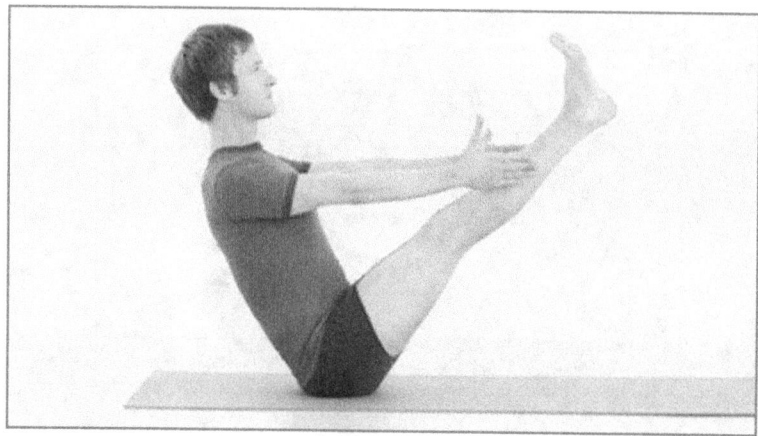

How To Do This Pose:

- Sit down on a yoga mat with your legs stretched out in front of you.
- Place your hands behind your back, making sure that your fingers are placed pointing towards your back.
- Then apply the slightest pressure on your hands and lean back a little, supporting your tailbone by sitting. Inhale as you do this.
- As you exhale lift up your legs until they are at a 45 degree angle off of the ground. Make sure that you do not bend your knees as you do this.
- Slowly release your arms and stretch them out in front of you. Make sure that your hands are parallel to the floor as you do so.
- With your legs and back off of the floor, you will remember the shape of a boat. Return to your beginning position and repeat.
- Continue with this pose for a duration of 30 seconds.

- If you suffer from high blood pressure or have suffered a hip injury in the past, you should avoid practicing this pose.

Pose 18. The Cobra Pose

The Cobra pose was originally created to help tone up the muscles in your upper back. This pose also helps to improve overall digestion and can even help alleviate breathing problems.

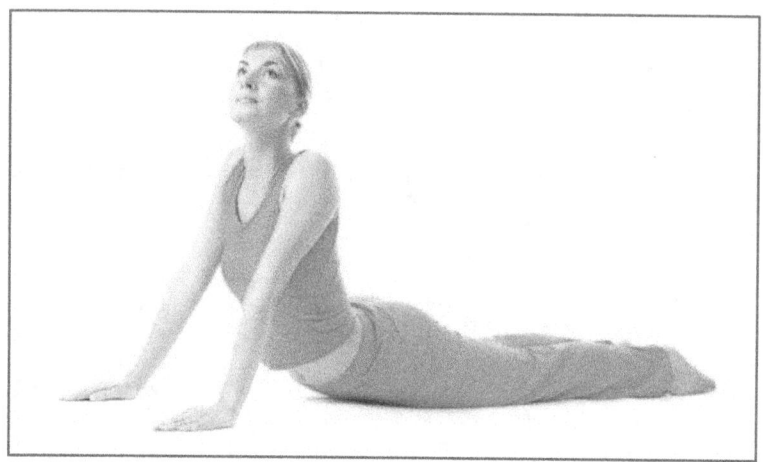

How To Do This Pose:

- Using a yoga mat, lie down flat on your stomach. Then place your palms close to your chest.
- As you inhale, slowly lift both your head and chest off of the floor.
- Then slowly rise even further, making sure that your hands are fully stretched out. Only lift up your hands as far as your abdomen. Make sure that you do not lift your hips off of the floor.
- Then pull your shoulders back, making sure that your chest is expanded. Make sure that you look straight ahead.
- Return to your beginning position.
- Continue with this pose for a duration of 20 seconds.
- If you are someone who suffers from carpal tunnel syndrome, hernia, or high blood pressure, do not do the Cobra Pose.

Pose 19. The Classic Locust Pose

This pose is used in such a way that it will strengthen your lower back and your abdominal muscles at the same time. This is one pose that is highly effective for sciatica.

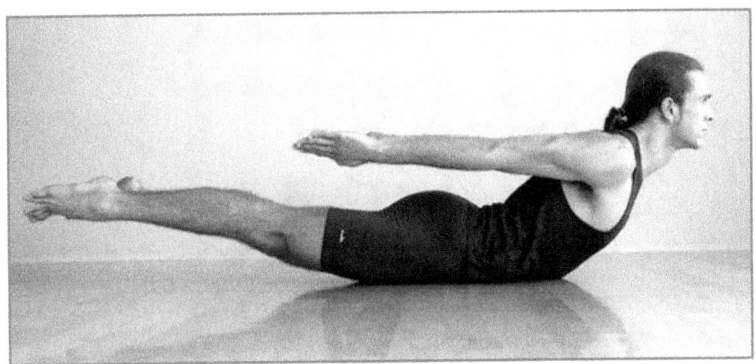

How To Do This Pose:

- The first thing that you will want to do is lie down on a yoga mat flat onto your stomach. Place your hands by your sides and place your chin on the floor.
- As you inhale and then slowly exhale, lift both of your legs off of the floor. Lift them as high as you possibly can. Make sure that you do not bend your knees.
- Return to the beginning position and repeat.
- Continue with this pose for a duration of 20 seconds.
- If you are suffering from chronic neck and back pain, I highly recommend that you avoid trying this pose.

Pose 20. The Bow Pose

The bow pose helps not only to strengthen your back, but it will also help to reduce the amount of belly fat that you have. This pose can also help alleviate constipation and aids in digestion.

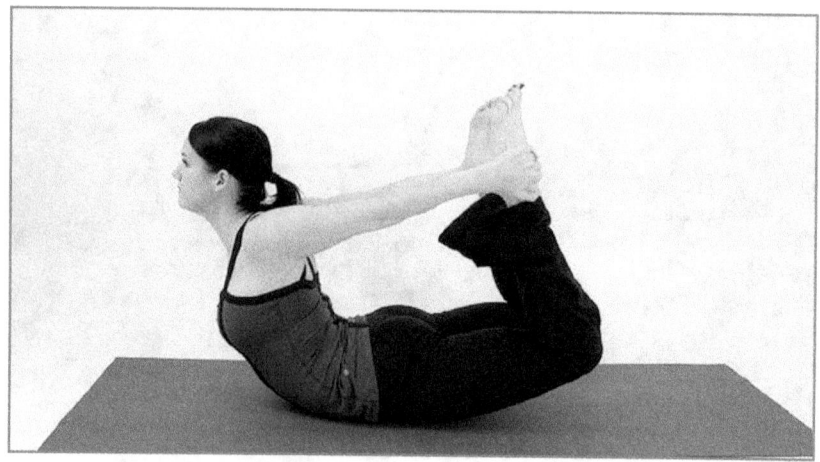

How To Do This Pose:

- Using your yoga mat, lie down flat on your stomach. Make sure that you bend both of your legs and grab a hold of both of your ankles.
- As you inhale, lift both your chest and thighs off of the ground and exhale as your rest onto your abdomen. Remember, the more that you lift off of the ground, the better arch you will have on your spine.
- Return to your beginning position and repeat.
- Continue the pose for a duration of 20 seconds.
- If you suffer from chronic back issues, I recommend that you only practice this pose under the supervision of an experienced instructor.

Pose 21. The Crocodile Pose

Just as the name implies, this pose is used primarily as a relaxation pose, which makes it excellent for those suffering from back problems. It can also help to treat high blood pressure in many cases.

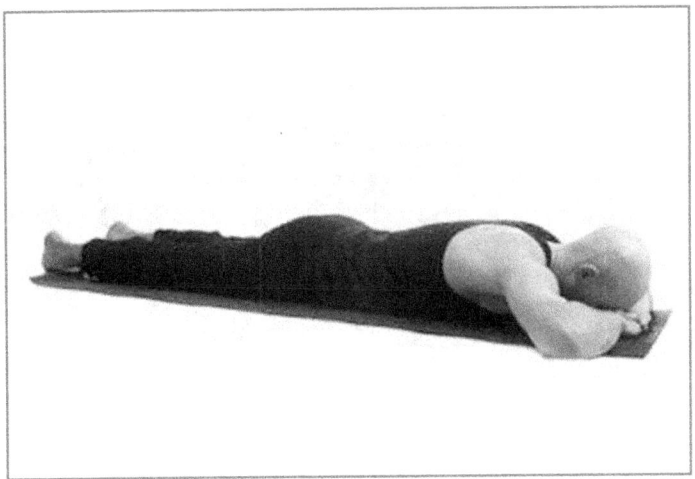

How To Do This Pose:

- The first thing that you will want to do is lie flat on your stomach upon your yoga mat. Make sure that you leave your legs apart and completely relaxed with your toes pointing out.
- Then place your right palm over your left hand and your left palm on the ground under your right hand.
- Then place your forehead onto your right hand, right at the bend of your hand. If you want to, also try folding your hands with your forehead placed upon them.
- Next close your eyes and completely relax your entire body. Make sure that you inhale and exhale.
- Do this pose for a duration of 3 to 5 minutes. However, if you want to relax longer, feel free to do so.

Pose 22. The Fish Pose

This is one pose that you can use to relieve any back or neck pain that you may be having. It also helps to alleviate constipation as well as increase your overall lung capacity, which can help to alleviate asthma or other breathing ailments.

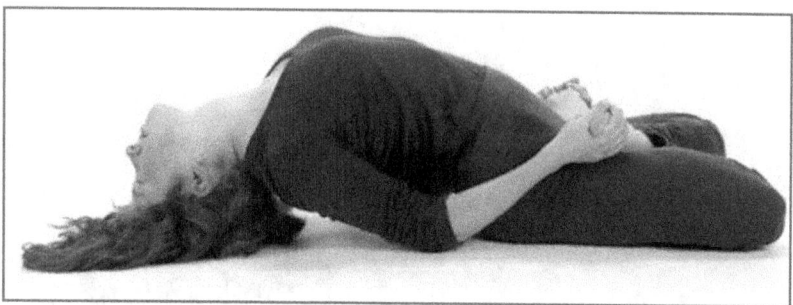

How To Do This Pose:

- The first thing that you will want to do is sit in the lotus position.
- Then place your right elbow on the ground, making sure that you are bending backwards. At the same time place your left elbow onto the ground just behind your back. Lie down upon the floor with your legs crossed.
- The next thing that you will want to do is to bring your hands over your head and place your arms on the floor behind you. Make sure that your fingers are pointed towards your shoulders.
- When you place your palms down, lift your head and arch your back. Place your head on the floor. As you do this make sure that you inhale.
- Hold onto your toes with your fingers. At the same time stretch out your leg and keep your palms on your thighs the entire time.
- Return to your lying position and before you decide to get up, perform the corpse pose.
- Continue to do the pose for a duration to 2 to 3 minutes.

- If you are suffering from severe neck and back problems, make sure that you use blocks to support your back. If you are suffering from high or low blood pressure, make sure that when you practice this pose to do so under supervision from a yoga instructor.

Pose 23. The Hand to Feet Pose

This is one of the best poses to do if you are looking to stretch out your entire body. It will help to tone up the muscles in your shoulder, abdomen, knees, hips, and thighs. This is one of the best poses to use it you are looking to treat sciatic conditions.

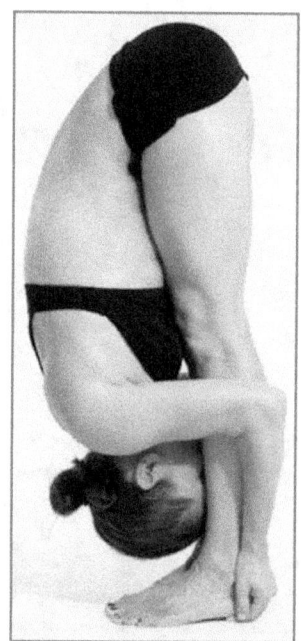

How To Do This Pose:

- The first thing that you will want to do is to stand straight up with your feet placed close together.
- As you inhale, lift your arms up over your head and then bend slightly backwards.
- As you exhale bend your body forward and bring your hands down to the sides of your feet. Feel free to bring your hands just behind your feet and place your fingers just underneath your heels.
- Return to your beginning position and repeat.

- Continue this pose for a duration of 20 seconds.
- If you are suffering from spinal problems and high blood pressure, I do not recommend that you do this pose.

Pose 24. The Half Waist Wheel Pose

This is one of the best poses to do if you are suffering from breathing problems. This pose will help to improve lung capacity and alleviate some respiratory symptoms such as asthma or COPD. It will also help to reduce excess fat from the waistline.

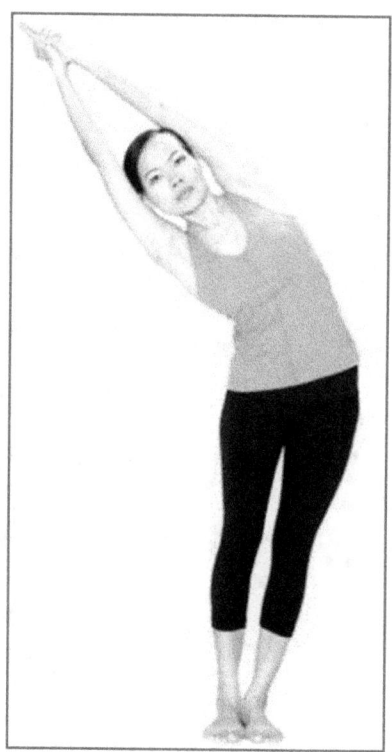

How To Do This Pose:

- Stand up straight with your feet placed close together.
- Then lift your left hand over your head, letting your biceps remain close to your ear.
- As you exhale bend your body towards the right. Make sure that you let your hand be stretched out, making sure that you do not bend your elbow as you do so. Or you can also raise both of your

hands over your head, lock your fingers together, and bend towards the right with your elbows stretched out.

- Return to the beginning position and repeat the same process in the opposite direction.
- Continue the pose for a duration of 20 seconds.
- Remember, while you bend, bend perfectly without going either forward or backward.

Pose 25. The Chair Pose

This is one of the best poses to do if you are looking to trim away excess of fat by strengthen your spinal cord and legs. It will also help to improve your overall immunity, making you feel much healthier than you may have previously felt.

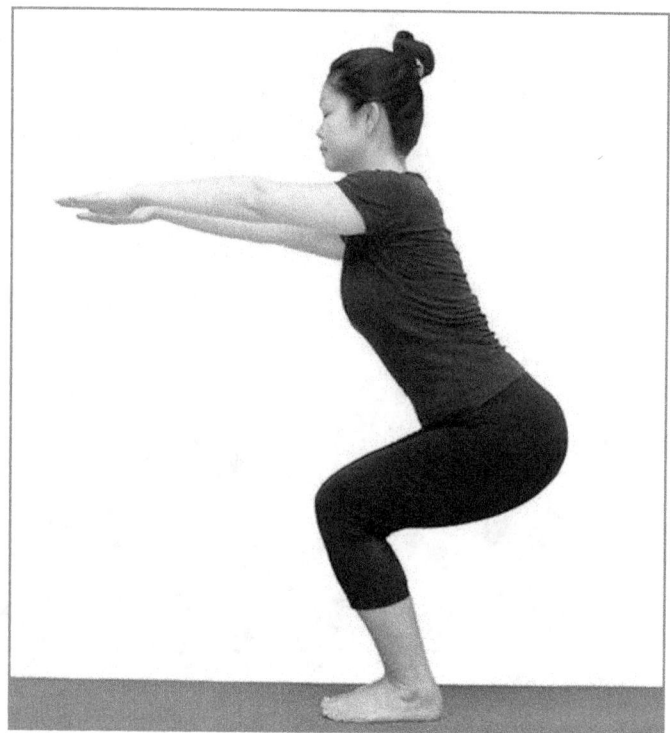

How To Do This Pose:

- Stand straight up with your feet held slightly apart.
- Then stretch out your hands in front of you, making sure that you keep them at level with your shoulders.
- As you exhale, squat your body as if you are sitting on a chair. Make sure that you do not bend forward. As you do this, straighten your back and try to keep it as perfectly straight as possible.

- Return to the beginning position and repeat.
- Continue to do this pose for a duration of 30 seconds.
- If you are suffering from low blood pressure or are suffering from insomnia, I do not recommend that you try this pose.

Pose 26. The Triangle Pose

The Triangle Pose not only helps to improve overall digestion, but it can help reduce excess fat that may be accumulating around your hip area. This will also help to strengthen your legs and spinal column.

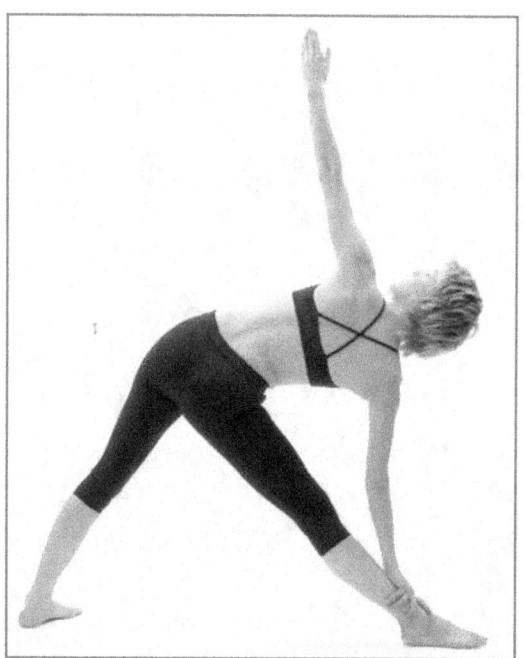

How To Do This Pose:

- The first thing that you will want to do is stand straight up with at least a distance of two feet between your feet.
- As you inhale, lift your hands at your side until they are level with your shoulders.
- As you exhale, bend towards the right, making sure that you hold your right ankle with your right hand.
- Then, as you bend towards the right, lift up your left arm up until it aligns with your left shoulder.
- Turn your head and stare at the thumb of your left arm.

- Return to the beginning position and repeat the process in the opposite direction.
- Continue to do this pose for a duration of 30 seconds.
- If you are suffering from low blood pressure or high blood pressure I do not recommend that you try this pose for yourself. If you are suffering from some kind of neck condition, try to avoid turning your head up. Just look straight in this instance.

Pose 27. The Mountain Pose

The Mountain Pose is the foundation for all of the standing postures and improves posture, groundedness, stability and confidence.

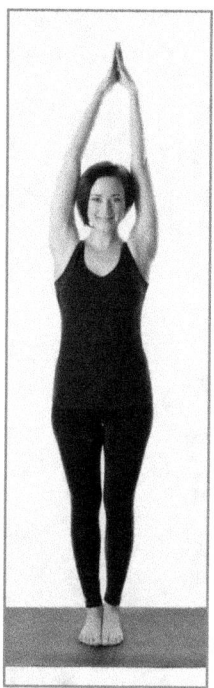

How To Do This Pose:

- From a standing position, place your feet together. Lift up the toes, spread them wide and place them back on the floor. Feel your weight evenly balanced through the bottom of each foot, not leaning forward or back.
- Flex an squeeze the your thighs and tuck your tailbone slightly under. Feel your hips aligned directly over the ankles. Keep your legs straight, but do not lock your knees.
- Inhale and lift your chest out of the waist, stretching your head up towards the ceiling, feeling the spine long and straight.

- Exhale and drop your shoulders down as you reach your fingertips towards the floor. Gently press your chest/sternum towards the front of the room.
- Continuing to reach out through your fingers, inhale and bring your arms straight up and place palms together up above your head.
- Exhale and relax the shoulders down from the ears while still reaching up.
- Breathe in once again and hold for a few seconds. Repeat with 4-8 breaths.
- Then, exhale and bring your arms back down to your sides.

Pose 28. The Tree Pose

This is one pose that is meant to improve your balance, making it perfect for those who refer to themselves as clumsy. This pose will strengthen your spin and help to combat aging.

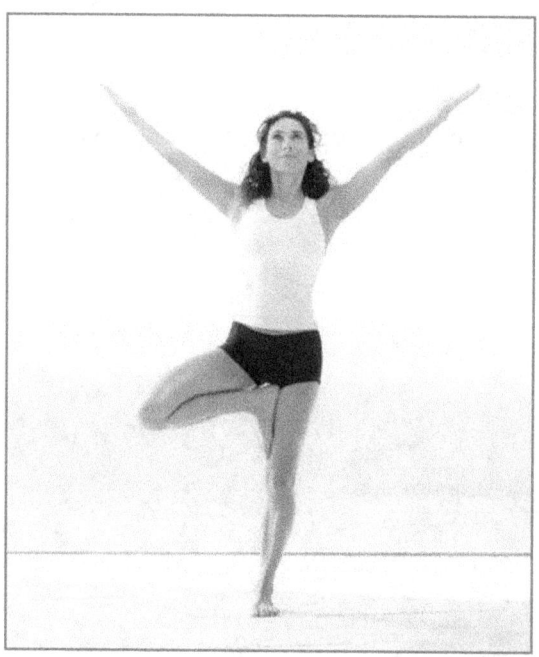

How To Do This Pose:

- The first thing that you will want to do is stand straight up with your hands placed at your sides.
- Then bend your right leg and place your right foot against your left inner thigh. The heel of your foot should touch the top of your inner thigh, making sure to keep your toes pointing downwards.
- As you inhale, stretch out both of your hands at your sides and lift them high over your head.

- Exhale and bring your palms together, stretching your hands out as much as possible. Make sure that you do not bend your elbows in the process.
- Keep your eyes fixed straight.
- Return to the beginning position and repeat the process with your other leg.
- Continue to do this pose for a duration of 30 seconds.
- People who are suffering from severe knee and hip issues and those struggling with insomnia should avoid practicing this pose at all costs.

Pose 29. The Warrior Pose

This pose is called the Warrior pose for a reason simply because you will feel like one as you do it. This pose will help to strengthen your lung function and with strengthen your legs in the process. This pose will also help to alleviate any back pain that you may have.

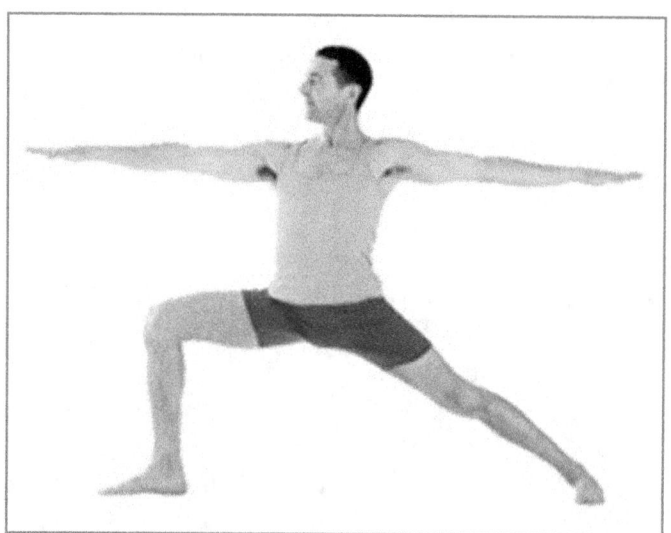

How To Do This Pose:

- The first thing that you will want to do is stand straight up with your fee placed apart from one another. Make sure that you keep a distance of about 4 feet in between your feet.
- Then turn your right foot out at a 90 degree angle. Then turn your left foot slowly towards the right.
- With your feet placed firmly onto the floor, exhale and turn the upper part of your body towards the right.
- Bend your leg so that your right thigh is parallel to the ground and your right knee is perfectly aligned with your right foot.
- Next, stretch your arms sideways and high until they are level with your shoulders.

- Return to the beginning position and repeat the pose in the opposite direction.
- Continue to do this pose for a duration of 30 seconds.
- If you are suffering from high blood pressure I do not recommend that you do this pose whatsoever. If you are suffering from severe neck pain, do not look to the side. Instead keep your gaze fixed straight ahead.

Pose 30. The Corpse Pose

This pose is used to help relax the entire body. It will help to rejuvenate the mind which is great for people who are under a lot of stress of who have trouble sleeping at night.

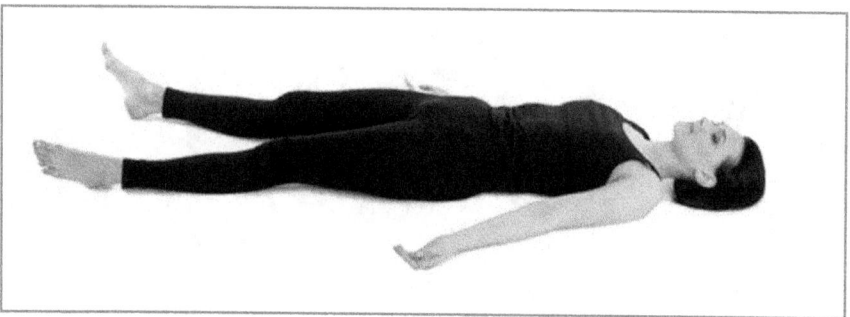

How To Do This Pose:

- The first thing that you will want to do is to lie flat on your back upon a yoga mat. Place your legs slightly apart from one another and keep your hands slightly away from your body.
- Close your eyes and keep in mind that all of the parts of your body are completely relaxed. As you do this, slowly inhale and exhale to relax fully.
- Feel free to remain in this pose for as long as you want. This is one pose that should be performed at the end of every yoga session that you have.

Conclusion

Thank you again for purchasing this yoga book!

I hope that by learning about the history and health benefits of yoga, it will show you how beneficial yoga can be for you. Remember, yoga is more than just an art form. Yoga is a way of life. There are many health benefits of yoga that will not only benefit you physically, but mentally and spiritually as well.

In this book, you have found specific instruction on how to do various yoga poses that shouldn't be too difficult for the beginner yoga practitioner. As long as you remember to breathe as you go through the poses and remember to not push yourself too hard, yoga will benefit you in a variety of ways that you never thought possible.

Once you get used to yoga, you will become a yoga master in no time. Good luck!

Before you go, would you please do me a favor? As an Independent Author and Self-Publisher, I don't have a large publishing company promoting my books. What I do have though, are reviews from readers like you. In fact, reviews are the single most important way for me to be able to get in front of more readers. Without them, I have no chance in competing with the larger, more established authors.

With that said, would you please go back and leave an honest review for this book? I would sincerely appreciate it.